Mediterranean Diet Cookbook

The complete guide with the best, easy and healthy recipes, improve your lifestyle now.

Marta Anderson

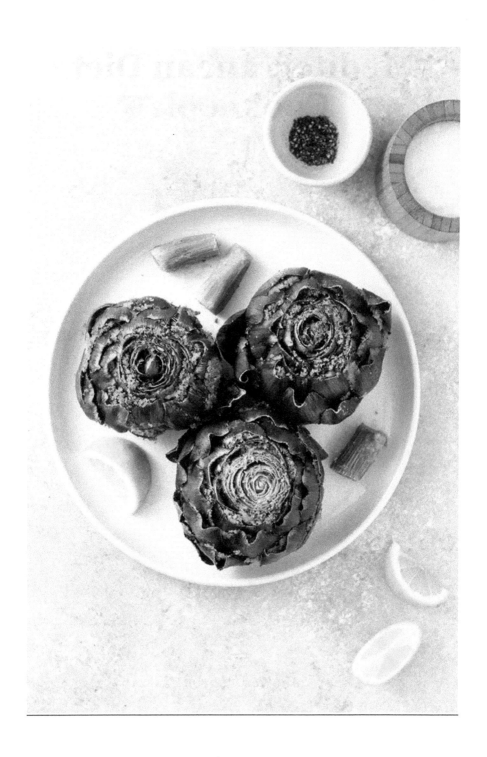

The information in the following pages is broadly considered a truthful and accurate account of facts and as such, any inattention, use, or misuse of the information in question by the reader will render any resulting actions solely under their purview. There are no scenarios in which the publisher or the original author of this work can be in any fashion deemed liable for any hardship or damages that may befall them after undertaking information described herein.

Additionally, the information in the following pages is intended only for informational purposes and should thus be thought of as universal. As befitting its nature, it is presented without assurance regarding its prolonged validity or interim quality. Trademarks that are mentioned are done without written consent and can in no way be considered an endorsement from the trademark holder.

Introduction:

What is Mediterranean Diet?

The Mediterranean Diet is a Diet Inspired by the Eating Habits of Spain, Italy, and Greece in the 1960s. In this Book you will Find Everything You Need to Cook Healthy and Delicious Recipes. All the Ingredients will be Easy to Find and You will be Followed Step By Step for the Realization of the Recipes

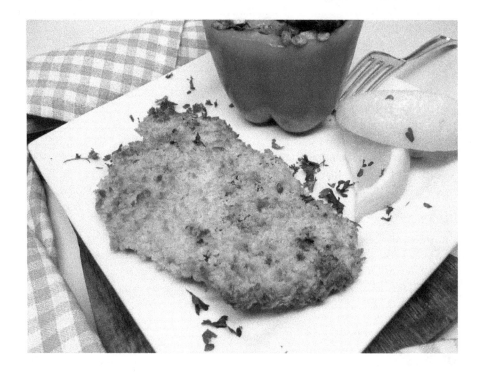

Table of Contents

Snacks

Smoked Salmon and Cheese on Rye Bread

Preparation Time: 15 minutes

Cooking Time: 10 minutes

Servings: 4

Ingredients:

- 8 ounces (250 g) smoked salmon, thinly sliced

- 1/3 cup (85 g) mayonnaise

- 2 tablespoons (30 ml) lemon juice

- 1 tablespoon (15 g) Dijon mustard

- 1 teaspoon (3 g) garlic, minced

- 4 slices cheddar cheese (about 2 oz. or 30 g each)

- 8 slices rye bread (about 2 oz. or 30 g each)

- 8 (15 g) Romaine lettuce leaves

- Salt and freshly ground black pepper

Directions:

1. Mix together the mayonnaise, lemon juice, mustard, and garlic in a small bowl. Flavor with salt and pepper and set aside.

2. Spread dressing on 4 bread slices. Top with lettuce, salmon, and cheese. Cover with remaining rye bread slices.

3. Serve and enjoy.

Nutrition:

Calories: 365

Fat: 16.6 g

Carbohydrates: 31.6 g

Protein: 18.8 g

Sodium: 951 mg

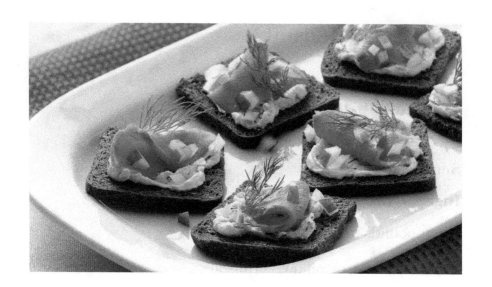

Pan-Fried Trout

Preparation Time: 15 minutes

Cooking Time: 10 minutes

Servings: 4

Ingredients:

- 1 ¼ pounds trout fillets

- 1/3 cup white, or yellow, cornmeal

- ¼ teaspoon anise seeds

- ¼ teaspoon black pepper

- ½ cup minced cilantro, or parsley

- Vegetable cooking spray

- Lemon wedges

Directions:

1. Coat fish with combined cornmeal, spices, and cilantro, pressing it gently into fish. Spray large skillet with cooking spray; heat over medium heat until hot.

2. Add fish and cook until fish is tender and flakes with fork, about 5 minutes on each side. Serve with lemon wedges.

Nutrition:

Calories: 207

Total Carbohydrate: 19 g

Cholesterol: 27 mg

Total Fat: 16 g

Fiber: 4 g

Protein: 18g

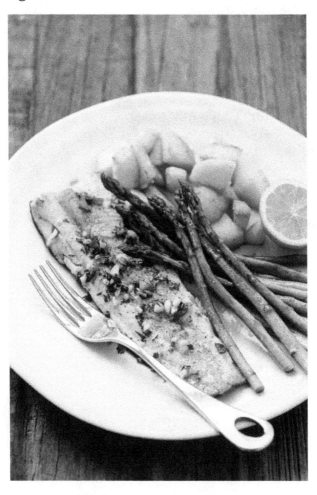

Greek Tuna Salad Bites

Preparation Time: 5 Minutes

Cooking Time: 10 Minutes

Servings: 6

Ingredients:

- Cucumbers (2 medium)

- White tuna (2 - 6 oz. cans.)

- Lemon juice (half of 1 lemon)

- Red bell pepper (.5 cup)

- Sweet/red onion (.25 cup)

- Black olives (.25 cup)

- Garlic (2 tablespoon.)

- Olive oil (2 tablespoon.)

- Fresh parsley (2 tablespoon.)

- Dried oregano - salt & pepper (as desired)

Directions:

1. Drain and flake the tuna. Juice the lemon. Dice/chop the onions, olives, pepper, parsley, and garliCup Slice each of the cucumbers into thick rounds (skin off or on).

2. In a mixing container, combine the rest of the fixings.

3. Place a heaping spoonful of salad onto the rounds and enjoy for your next party or just a snack.

Nutrition:

Calories: 400

Fats: 22 g

Carbs: 26 g

Fiber Content: 8 g

Protein: 30 g

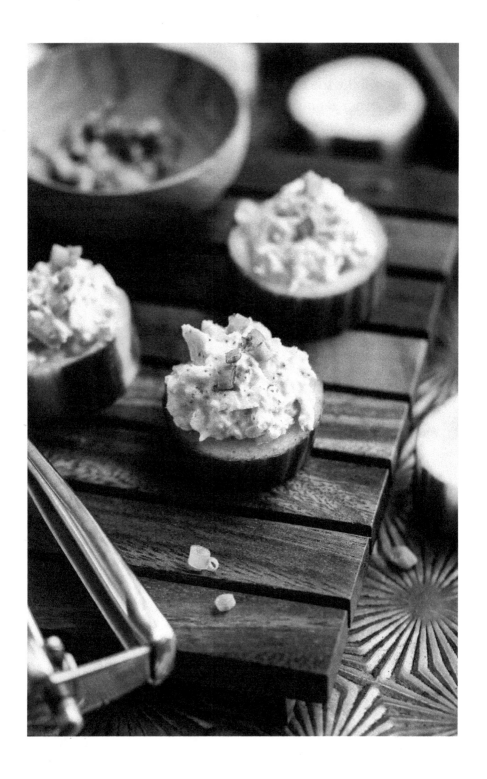

Veggie Fritters

Preparation Time: 10 minutes

Cooking Time: 10 minutes

Servings: 4

Ingredients:

- 2 garlic cloves, minced

- 2 yellow onions, chopped

- 4 scallions, chopped

- 2 carrots, grated

- 2 teaspoons cumin, ground

- ½ teaspoon turmeric powder

- Salt and black pepper to the taste

- ¼ teaspoon coriander, ground

- 2 tablespoons parsley, chopped

- ¼ teaspoon lemon juice

- ½ cup almond flour

- 2 beets, peeled and grated

- 2 eggs, whisked

- ¼ cup tapioca flour

- 3 tablespoons olive oil

Directions:

1. In a bowl, combine the garlic with the onions, scallions and the rest of the ingredients except the oil, stir well and shape medium fritters out of this mix.

2. Heat up a pan with the oil over medium-high heat, add the fritters, cook for 5 minutes on each side, arrange on a platter and serve.

Nutrition:

Calories 209;

Fat 11.2 g;

Fiber 3 g;

Carbs 4.4 g;

Protein 4.8 g

White Bean Dip

Preparation Time: 10 minutes

Cooking Time: 0 minute

Servings: 4

Ingredients:

- 15 ounces canned white beans, drained and rinsed

- 6 ounces canned artichoke hearts, drained and quartered

- 4 garlic cloves, minced

- 1 tablespoon basil, chopped

- 2 tablespoons olive oil

- Juice of ½ lemon

- Zest of ½ lemon, grated

- Salt and black pepper to the taste

Directions:

1. In your food processor, combine the beans with the artichokes and the rest of the ingredients except the oil and pulse well.

2. Add the oil gradually, pulse the mix again, divide into cups and serve as a party dip.

Nutrition:

Calories 274;

Fat 11.7 g;

Fiber 6.5 g;

Carbs 18.5 g;

Protein 16.5 g

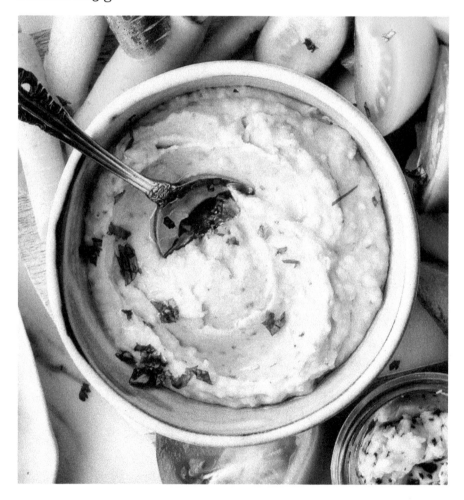

Eggplant Dip

Preparation Time: 10 minutes

Cooking Time: 40 minutes

Servings: 4

Ingredients:

- 1 eggplant, poked with a fork

- 2 tablespoons tahini paste

- 2 tablespoons lemon juice

- 2 garlic cloves, minced

- 1 tablespoon olive oil

- Salt and black pepper to the taste

- 1 tablespoon parsley, chopped

Directions:

1. Put the eggplant in a roasting pan, bake at 400° F for 40 minutes, cool down, peel and transfer to your food processor.

2. Add the rest of the ingredients except the parsley, pulse well, divide into small bowls and serve as an appetizer with the parsley sprinkled on top.

Nutrition:

Calories 121;

Fat 4.3 g;

Fiber 1 g;

Carbs 1.4 g;

Protein 4.3 g

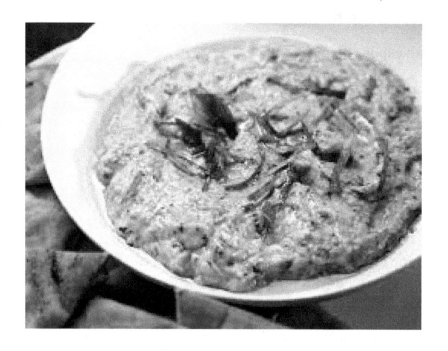

Bulgur Lamb Meatballs

Preparation Time: 10 minutes

Cooking Time: 15 minute

Servings: 6

Ingredients:

- 1 and ½ cups Greek yogurt
- ½ teaspoon cumin, ground
- 1 cup cucumber, shredded
- ½ teaspoon garlic, minced
- A pinch of salt and black pepper
- 1 cup bulgur
- 2 cups water
- 1 pound lamb, ground
- ¼ cup parsley, chopped
- ¼ cup shallots, chopped
- ½ teaspoon allspice, ground
- ½ teaspoon cinnamon powder
- 1 tablespoon olive oil

Directions:

1. In a bowl, combine the bulgur with the water, cover the bowl, leave aside for 10 minutes, drain and transfer to a bowl.

2. Add the meat, the yogurt and the rest of the ingredients except the oil, stir well and shape medium meatballs out of this mix.

3. Heat up a pan with the oil over medium-high heat, add the meatballs, cook them for 7 minutes on each side, arrange them all on a platter and serve as an appetizer.

Nutrition:

Calories 300;

Fat 9.6 g;

Fiber 4.6 g;

Carbs 22.6 g;

Protein 6.6 g

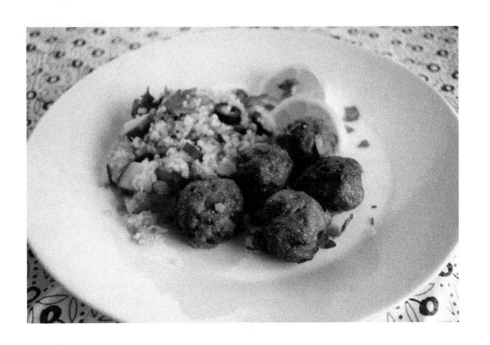

Poultry

Buffalo Wings

Preparation Time: 5 minutes

Cooking Time: 12 minutes

Servings: 4

Ingredients:

- 2 pounds (907 g) chicken wings, patted dry

- 1 teaspoon seasoned salt

- ¼ teaspoon pepper

- ½ teaspoon garlic powder

- ¼ cup buffalo sauce

- 3/4 cup chicken broth

- 1/3 cup blue cheese crumbles

- ¼ cup cooked bacon crumbles

- 2 stalks green onion, sliced

Directions:

1. Season the chicken wings with salt, pepper, and garlic powder.

2. Pour the buffalo sauce and broth into the Instant Pot. Stir in the chicken wings.

3. Lock the lid. Select the Manual mode and set the cooking time for 12 minutes at High Pressure.

4. Once cooking is complete, do a quick pressure release. Carefully open the lid. Gently stir to coat wings with the sauce.

5. If you prefer crispier wings, you can broil them for 3 to 5 minutes until the skin is crispy.

6. Remove the chicken wings from the pot to a plate. Brush them with the leftover sauce and serve topped with the blue cheese, bacon, and green onions.

Nutrition:

calories: 536

fat: 37.3g

protein: 47.1g

carbs: 1.0g

net carbs: 0.8g

fiber: 0.2g

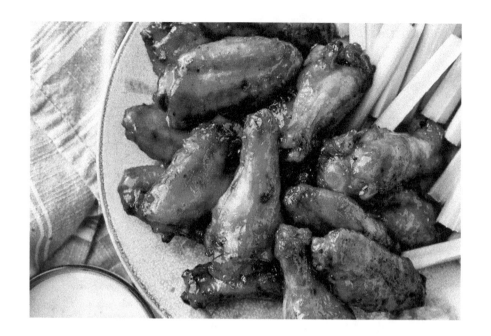

Sesame Chicken

Preparation Time: 5 minutes

Cooking Time: 24 minutes

Servings: 4

Ingredients:

- 1 pound (454 g) boneless, skinless chicken thighs, cut into bite-sized pieces and patted dry

- Fine sea salt, to taste

- 2 tablespoons avocado oil or coconut oil

- 1 clove garlic, smashed to a paste

- ½ cup chicken broth

- 1/2 cup coconut aminos

- 1/3 cup Swerve

- 2 tablespoons toasted sesame oil

- 1 tablespoon lime juice

- ¼ teaspoon peeled and grated fresh ginger

For Garnish:

- Sesame seeds

- Sliced green onions

Directions:

1. Season all sides of chicken thighs with salt.

2. Set your Instant Pot to Sauté and heat the avocado oil.

3. Add the chicken thighs and sear for about 4 minutes, or until lightly browned on all sides.

4. Remove the chicken and set aside.

5. Add the remaining ingredients to the Instant Pot and cook for 10 minutes, stirring occasionally, or until the sauce is reduced and thickened.

6. Return the chicken thighs to the pot and cook for 10 minutes, stirring occasionally, or until the chicken is cooked through.

7. Sprinkle the sesame seeds and green onions on top for garnish and serve.

Nutrition:

calories: 359

fat: 29.3g

protein: 20.5g

carbs: 3.1g

net carbs: 3.0g

fiber: 1.0g

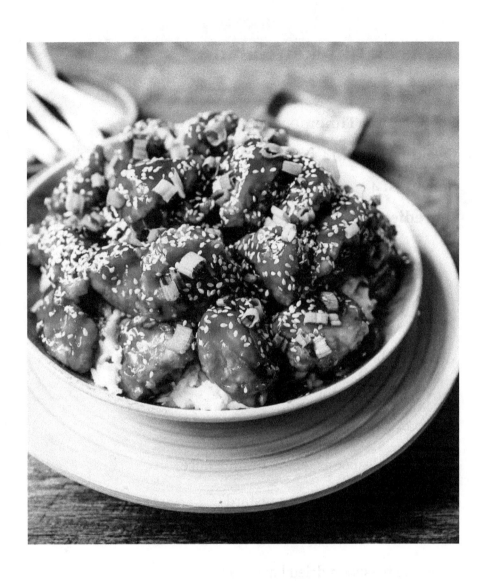

Greek Chicken Salad

Preparation Time: 10 minutes

Cooking Time: 14 minutes

Servings: 4

Ingredients:

- 4 bone-in, skin-on chicken thighs
- 1 teaspoon fine sea salt
- ¾ teaspoon ground black pepper
- 2 tablespoons unsalted butter
- 2 cloves garlic, minced
- ¼ cup red wine vinegar
- 2 tablespoons lemon or lime juice
- 2 teaspoons Dijon mustard
- ½ teaspoon dried oregano leaves
- ½ teaspoon dried basil leaves

Greek Salad:

- 2 cups Greek olives, pitted
- 1 medium tomato, diced
- 1 medium cucumber, diced
- ¼ cup diced red onions

- 2 tablespoons extra-virgin olive oil

- 4 sprigs fresh oregano

- 1 cup crumbled feta cheese, for garnish

Directions:

1. Sprinkle the chicken thighs on all sides with the salt and pepper.

2. Set your Instant Pot to Sauté and melt the butter.

3. Add the chicken thighs to the Instant Pot, skin-side down. Add the garlic and sauté for 4 minutes until golden brown.

4. Turn the chicken thighs over and stir in the vinegar, lemon juice, mustard, oregano, and basil.

5. Secure the lid. Select the Manual mode and set the cooking time for 10 minutes at High Pressure.

6. Once cooking is complete, do a quick pressure release. Carefully open the lid.

7. Meanwhile, toss all the salad ingredients except the cheese in a large serving dish. When the chicken is finished, take ¼ cup of the liquid from the Instant Pot and stir into the salad.

8. Place the chicken on top of the salad and serve garnished with the cheese.

Nutrition:

calories: 581

fat: 44.3g

protein: 38.5g

carbs: 7.3g

net carbs: 6.0g

fiber: 1.3g

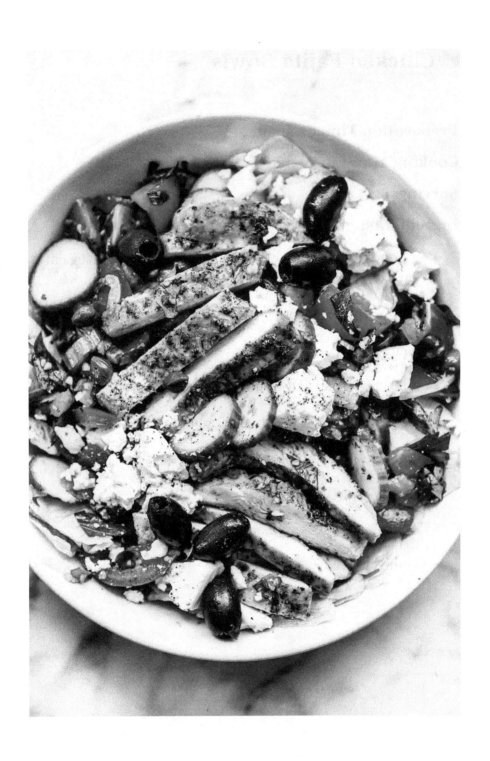

Chicken Fajita Bowls

Preparation Time: 5 minutes

Cooking Time: 10 minutes

Servings: 2

Ingredients:

- 1 pound (454 g) boneless, skinless chicken breasts, cut into 1-inch pieces

- 2 cups chicken broth

- 1 cup salsa

- 1 teaspoon paprika

- 1 teaspoon fine sea salt, or more to taste

- 1 teaspoon chili powder

- ½ teaspoon ground cumin

- ½ teaspoon ground black pepper

- 1 lime, halved

Directions:

1. Combine all the ingredients except the lime in the Instant Pot.

2. Lock the lid. Select the Manual mode and set the cooking time for 10 minutes at High Pressure.

3. When the timer beeps, perform a quick pressure release. Carefully remove the lid.

4. Shred the chicken with two forks and return to the Instant Pot. Squeeze the lime juice into the chicken mixture. Taste and add more salt, if needed. Give the mixture a good stir.

5. Ladle the chicken mixture into bowls and serve.

Nutrition:

calories: 281

fat: 6.3g

protein: 51.5g

carbs: 5.9g

net carbs: 4.9g

fiber: 1.0g

Prosciutto-Wrapped Chicken

Preparation Time: 5 minutes

Cooking Time: 15 minutes

Servings: 5

Ingredients:

- 1½ cups water
- 5 chicken breast halves, butterflied
- 2 garlic cloves, halved
- 1 teaspoon marjoram
- Sea salt, to taste
- ½ teaspoon red pepper flakes
- ¼ teaspoon ground black pepper, or more to taste
- 10 strips prosciutto

Directions:

1. Pour the water into the Instant Pot and insert the trivet.

2. Rub the chicken breast halves with garlic. Sprinkle with marjoram, salt, red pepper flakes, and black pepper. Wrap each chicken breast into 2 prosciutto strips and secure with toothpicks. Put the chicken on the trivet.

3. Lock the lid. Select the Poultry mode and set the cooking time for 15 minutes at High Pressure.

4. When the timer beeps, perform a natural pressure release for 10 minutes, then release any remaining pressure. Carefully remove the lid.

5. Remove the toothpicks and serve warm.

Nutrition:

calories: 550

fat: 28.6g

protein: 68.5g

carbs: 1.0g

net carbs: 0.8g

fiber: 0.2g

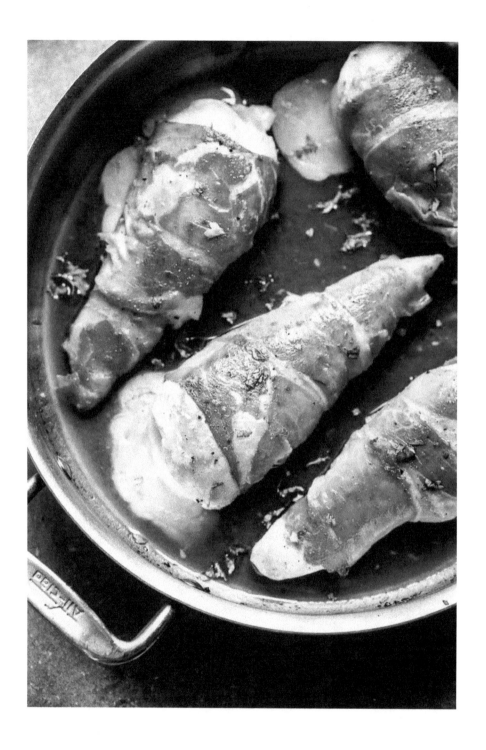

Creamy Chicken Cordon Bleu

Preparation Time: 12 minutes

Cooking Time: 15 minutes

Servings: 6

Ingredients:

- 4 boneless, skinless chicken breast halves, butterflied

- 4 (1-ounce / 28-g) slices Swiss cheese

- 8 (1-ounce / 28-g) slices ham

- 1 cup water

- Chopped fresh flat-leaf parsley, for garnish

Sauce:

- 1½ ounces (43 g) cream cheese (3 tablespoons)

- ¼ cup chicken broth

- 1 tablespoon unsalted butter

- ¼ teaspoon ground black pepper

- ¼ teaspoon fine sea salt

Directions:

1. Lay the chicken breast halves on a clean work surface. Top each with a slice of Swiss cheese and 2 slices of ham. Roll the chicken around the ham and cheese, then secure with toothpicks. Set aside.

2. Whisk together all the ingredients for the sauce in a small saucepan over medium heat, stirring until the cream cheese melts and the sauce is smooth.

3. Place the chicken rolls, seam-side down, in a casserole dish. Pour half of the sauce over the chicken rolls. Set the remaining sauce aside.

4. Pour the water into the Instant Pot and insert the trivet. Place the dish on the trivet.

5. Lock the lid. Select the Manual mode and set the cooking time for 15 minutes at High Pressure.

6. When the timer beeps, perform a natural pressure release for 10 minutes, then release any remaining pressure. Carefully remove the lid.

7. Remove the chicken rolls from the Instant Pot to a plate. Pour the remaining sauce over them and serve garnished with the parsley.

Nutrition:

calories: 314

fat: 13.6g

protein: 46.2g

carbs: 1.7g

net carbs: 1.7g

fiber: 0g

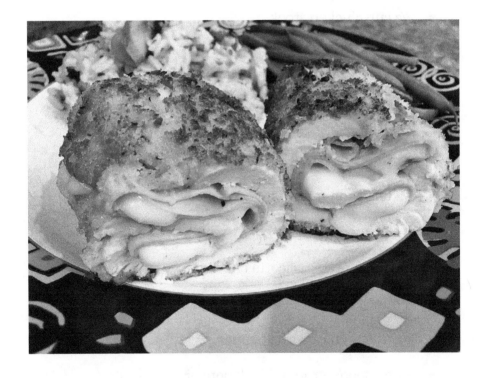

Cheesy Chicken Drumsticks

Preparation Time: 3 minutes

Cooking Time: 23 minutes

Servings: 5

Ingredients:

- 1 tablespoon olive oil

- 5 chicken drumsticks

- ½ cup chicken stock

- ¼ cup unsweetened coconut milk

- ¼ cup dry white wine

- 2 garlic cloves, minced

- 1 teaspoon shallot powder

- ½ teaspoon marjoram

- ½ teaspoon thyme

- 6 ounces (170 g) ricotta cheese

- 4 ounces (113 g) Cheddar cheese

- ½ teaspoon cayenne pepper

- ¼ teaspoon ground black pepper

- Sea salt, to taste

Directions:

1. Set your Instant Pot to Sauté and heat the olive oil until sizzling.

2. Add the chicken drumsticks and brown each side for 3 minutes.

3. Stir in the chicken stock, milk, wine, garlic, shallot powder, marjoram, thyme.

4. Lock the lid. Select the Manual mode and set the cooking time for 15 minutes at High Pressure.

5. When the timer beeps, perform a natural pressure release for 10 minutes, then release any remaining pressure. Carefully remove the lid.

6. Shred the chicken with two forks and return to the Instant Pot.

7. Set your Instant Pot to Sauté again and add the remaining ingredients and stir well.

8. Cook for another 2 minutes, or until the cheese is melted. Taste and add more salt, if desired. Serve immediately.

Nutrition:

calories: 413

fat: 24.3g

protein: 41.9g

carbs: 4.6g

net carbs: 4.0g

fiber: 0.6g

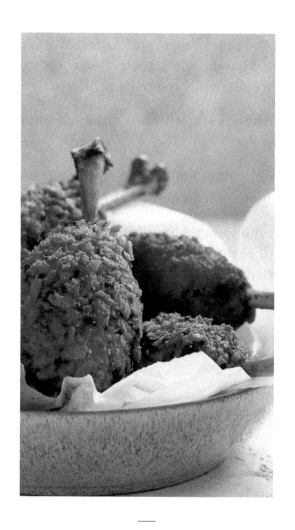

Sides

Cheddar Potato Gratin

Preparation Time: 15 minutes

Cooking Time: 20 minutes

Servings: 2

Ingredients:

- 2 potatoes
  - 1/3 cup half and half
  - 1 tablespoon oatmeal flour
  - ¼ teaspoon ground black pepper
  - 1 egg
- 2 oz. Cheddar cheese

Directions:

1. Wash the potatoes and slice them into thin pieces.

2. Preheat the air fryer to 365 F.

3. Put the potato slices in the air fryer and cook them for 10 minutes.

4. Meanwhile, combine the half and half, oatmeal flour, and ground black pepper.

5. Crack the egg into the liquid and whisk it carefully.

6. Shred Cheddar cheese.

7. When the potato is cooked – take 2 ramekins and place the potatoes on them.

8. Pour the half and half mixture.

9. Sprinkle the gratin with shredded Cheddar cheese.

10. Cook the gratin for 10 minutes at 360 F.

11. Serve the meal immediately.

12. Enjoy!

Nutrition:

Calories: 353

Fat: 16.6g

Fiber: 5.4g

Carbs: 37.2g

Protein: 15g

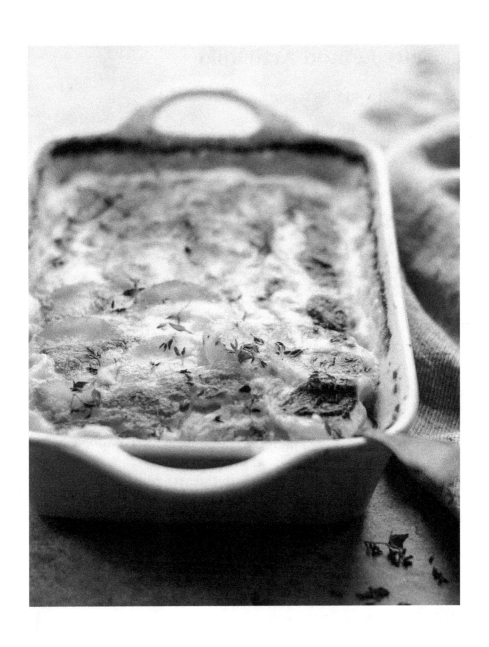

Salty Lemon Artichokes

Preparation Time: 15 minutes

Cooking Time: 45 minutes

Servings: 2

Ingredients:

- 1 lemon
- 2 artichokes
- 1 teaspoon kosher salt
- 1 garlic head
- 2 teaspoons olive oil

Directions:

1. Cut off the edges of the artichokes.

2. Cut the lemon into the halves.

3. Peel the garlic head and chop the garlic cloves roughly.

4. Then place the chopped garlic in the artichokes.

5. Sprinkle the artichokes with the olive oil and kosher salt.

6. Then squeeze the lemon juice into the artichokes.

7. Wrap the artichokes in the foil.

8. Preheat the air fryer to 330 F.

9. Place the wrapped artichokes in the air fryer and cook for 45 minutes.

10. When the artichokes are cooked – discard the foil and serve.

11. Enjoy!

Nutrition:

Calories: 133

Fat: 5g

Fiber: 9.7g

Carbs: 21.7g

Protein: 6g

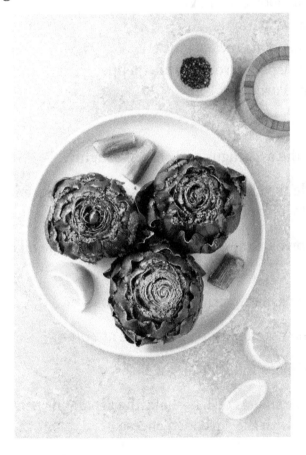

Asparagus & Parmesan

Preparation Time: 10 minutes

Cooking Time: 6 minutes

Servings: 2

Ingredients:

- 1 teaspoon sesame oil
- 11 oz. asparagus
- 1 teaspoon chicken stock
- ½ teaspoon ground white pepper
- 3 oz. Parmesan

Directions:

1. Wash the asparagus and chop it roughly.

2. Sprinkle the chopped asparagus with the chicken stock and ground white pepper.

3. Then sprinkle the vegetables with the sesame oil and shake them.

4. Place the asparagus in the air fryer basket.

5. Cook the vegetables for 4 minutes at 400 F.

6. Meanwhile, shred Parmesan cheese.

7. When the time is over – shake the asparagus gently and sprinkle with the shredded cheese.

8. Cook the asparagus for 2 minutes more at 400 F.

9. After this, transfer the cooked asparagus in the serving plates.

10. Serve and taste it!

Nutrition:

Calories: 189

Fat: 11.6g

Fiber: 3.4g

Carbs: 7.9g

Protein: 17.2g

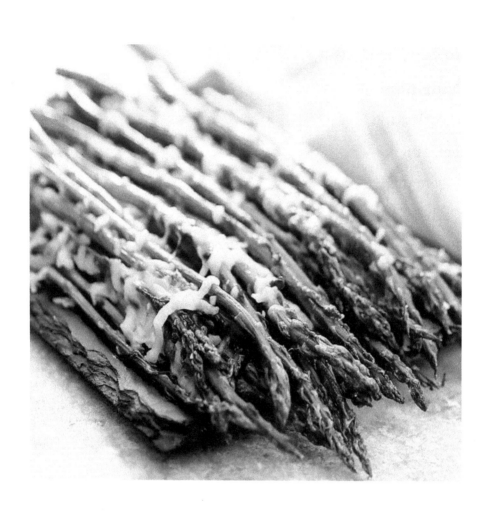

Carrot Lentil Burgers

Preparation Time: 10 minutes

Cooking Time: 12 minutes

Servings: 2

Ingredients:

- 6 oz. lentils, cooked
- 1 egg
- 2 oz. carrot, grated
- 1 teaspoon semolina
- ½ teaspoon salt
- 1 teaspoon turmeric
- 1 tablespoon butter

Directions:

1. Crack the egg into the bowl and whisk it.

2. Add the cooked lentils and mash the mixture with the help of the fork.

3. Then sprinkle the mixture with the grated carrot, semolina, salt, and turmeric.

4. Mix it up and make the medium burgers.

5. Put the butter into the lentil burgers. It will make them juicy.

6. Preheat the air fryer to 360 F.

7. Put the lentil burgers in the air fryer and cook for 12 minutes.

8. Flip the burgers into another side after 6 minutes of cooking.

9. Then chill the cooked lentil burgers and serve them.

10. Enjoy!

Nutrition:

Calories: 404

Fat: 9g

Fiber: 26.9g

Carbs: 56g

Protein: 25.3g

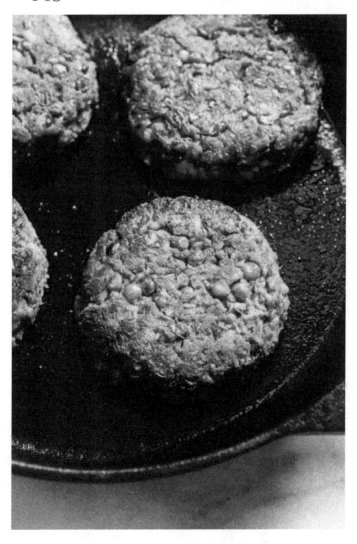

Corn on Cobs

Preparation Time: 10 minutes

Cooking Time: 10 minutes

Servings: 2

Ingredients:

- 2 fresh corn on cobs
- 2 teaspoon butter
- 1 teaspoon salt
- 1 teaspoon paprika
- ¼ teaspoon olive oil

Directions:

1. Preheat the air fryer to 400 F.

2. Rub the corn on cobs with the salt and paprika.

3. Then sprinkle the corn on cobs with the olive oil.

4. Place the corn on cobs in the air fryer basket.

5. Cook the corn on cobs for 10 minutes.

6. When the time is over – transfer the corn on cobs in the serving plates and rub with the butter gently.

7. Serve the meal immediately.

8. Enjoy!

Nutrition:

Calories: 122

Fat: 5.5g

Fiber: 2.4g

Carbs: 17.6g

Protein: 3.2g

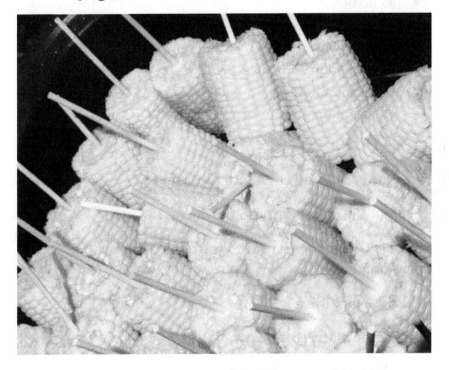

Sugary Carrot Strips

Preparation Time: 10 minutes

Cooking Time: 10 minutes

Servings: 2

Ingredients:

- 2 carrots
- 1 teaspoon brown sugar
- 1 teaspoon olive oil
- 1 tablespoon soy sauce
- 1 teaspoon honey
- ½ teaspoon ground black pepper

Directions:

1. Peel the carrot and cut it into the strips.

2. Then put the carrot strips in the bowl.

3. Sprinkle the carrot strips with the olive oil, soy sauce, honey, and ground black pepper.

4. Shake the mixture gently.

5. Preheat the air fryer to 360 F.

6. Cook the carrot for 10 minutes.

7. After this, shake the carrot strips well.

8. Enjoy!

Nutrition:

Calories: 67

Fat: 2.4g

Fiber: 1.7g

Carbs: 11.3g

Protein: 1.1g

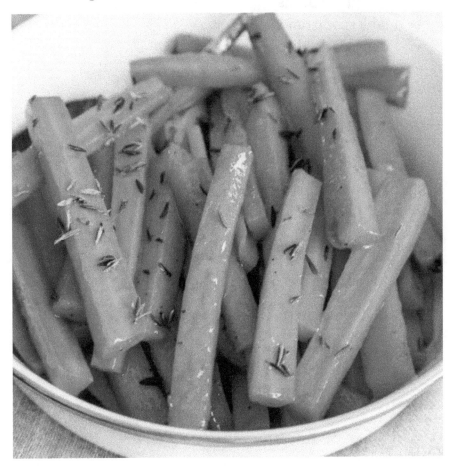

Onion Green Beans

Preparation Time: 10 minutes

Cooking Time: 12 minutes

Servings: 2

Ingredients:

- 11 oz. green beans
- 1 tablespoon onion powder
- 1 tablespoon olive oil
- ½ teaspoon salt
- ¼ teaspoon chili flakes

Directions:

1. Wash the green beans carefully and place them in the bowl.

2. Sprinkle the green beans with the onion powder, salt, chili flakes, and olive oil.

3. Shake the green beans carefully.

4. Preheat the air fryer to 400 F.

5. Put the green beans in the air fryer and cook for 8 minutes.

6. After this, shake the green beans and cook them for 4 minutes more at 400 F.

7. When the time is over – shake the green beans.

8. Serve the side dish and enjoy!

Nutrition:

Calories: 1205

Fat: 7.2g

Fiber: 5.5g

Carbs: 13.9g

Protein: 3.2g

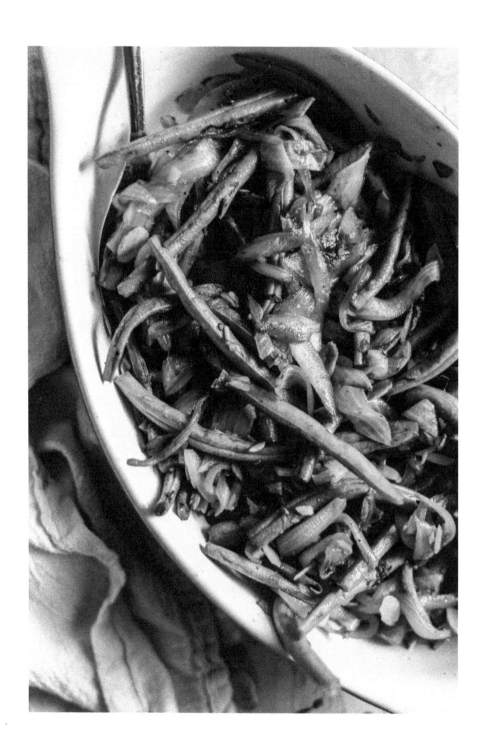

Desserts

Banana Bread

Preparation Time: 5 minutes

Cooking Time: 40 Minutes

Servings: 6

Ingredients:

- ¾ cup sugar

- 1/3 cup butter

- 1 tbsp. vanilla extract

- 1 egg

- 2 bananas

- 1 tbsp. baking powder

- 1 and ½ cups flour

- ½ tbsp. baking soda

- 1/3 cup milk

- 1 and ½ tbsp. cream of tartar

- Cooking spray

Directions:

1. Mix in milk with cream of tartar, vanilla, egg, sugar, bananas and butter in a bowl and turn whole.

2. Mix in flour with baking soda and baking powder.

3. Blend the 2 mixtures, turn properly, move into oiled pan with cooking spray, put into air fryer and cook at 320°F for 40 minutes.

4. Remove bread, allow to cool, slice.

5. Serve.

Nutrition:

Calories: 540

Total Fat: 16g

Total carbs: 28g

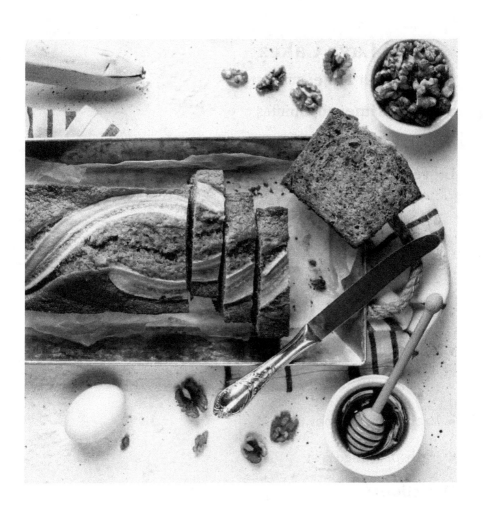

Mini Lava Cakes

Preparation Time: 5 minutes

Cooking Time: 20 Minutes

Servings: 3

Ingredients:

- 1 egg

- 4 tbsp. sugar

- 2 tbsp. olive oil

- 4 tbsp. milk

- 4 tbsp. flour

- 1 tbsp. cocoa powder

- ½ tbsp. baking powder

- ½ tbsp. orange zest

Directions:

1. Mix in egg with sugar, flour, salt, oil, milk, orange zest, baking powder and cocoa powder, turn properly. Move it to oiled ramekins.

2. Put ramekins in air fryer and cook at 320°F for 20 minutes.

3. Serve warm.

Nutrition:

Calories: 329

Total Fat: 8.5g

Total carbs: 12.4g

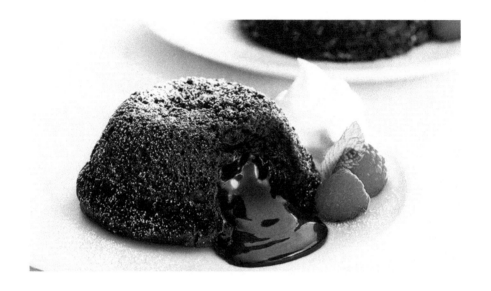

Lunch

Amazing Low Carb Shrimp Lettuce Wraps.

Preparation Time: 10 minutes

Cooking Time: 4 minutes

Servings: 4

Ingredients:

For Thai Shrimp:

- 1 lb of Shrimp, peeled, deveined
- 2 tablespoons of Coconut aminos
- 1/4 cup of Olive oil, divided
- 1 tablespoon of Fish sauce
- 2 teaspoons of Lime juice
- 1/4 teaspoon of Crushed red pepper flakes

For Lettuce Wraps:

- 16 leaves of Bibb lettuce
- 1/3 fresh Cucumber, julienned
- 1 Avocado, diced

For Peanut Sauce:

- 1/4 cup of Peanut butter

- 1/4 cup of Coconut aminos

- 1 1/2 tablespoon of Lime juice

- 1/2 teaspoon of Crushed red pepper flakes

- 1/4 teaspoon of Sea salt

- 1/4 teaspoon of Garlic powder

For Garnish: Sliced green onions, lime wedges, roasted peanuts

Directions:

1. Combine two tablespoons of olive oil, coconut aminos, fish sauce, red peppers, and lime juice in a bowl.

2. Add in the shrimp and stir to mix. Cover the bowl and keep aside to marinate for thirty minutes.

3. Combine the peanut sauce **Ingredients:** and keep aside. Pour two tablespoons of oil into a pan and place over medium heat.

4. Add in shrimp and cook until opaque, about six minutes. Share the cucumbers, shrimp, and avocados among the lettuce leaves. Add in a drizzle of peanut sauce and garnish with peanuts, green onions, and lime wedges if desired.

Nutrition:

Servings: 4 lettuce wraps

Calories: 470

Protein: 29g

Fat: 31g

Carbohydrates: 16g

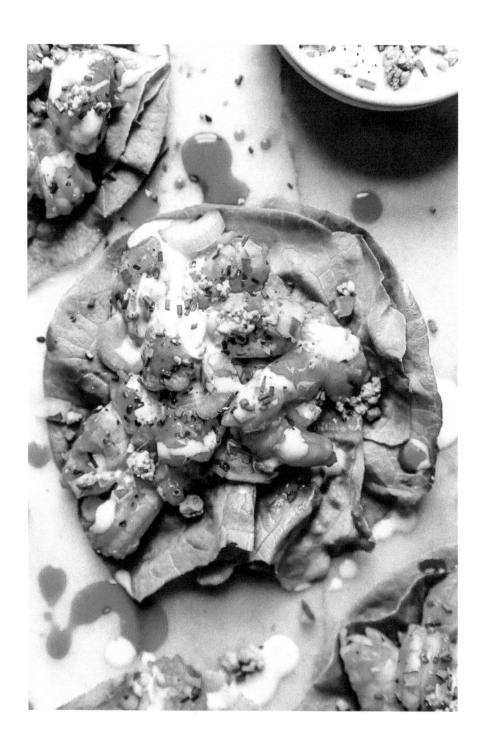

Tasty Low Carb Cucumber Salad.

Preparation Time: 10 minutes

Cooking Time: 0 minutes

Servings: 6

Ingredients:

- 1/2 cup of Sour cream
- 2 tablespoons of Fresh dill, chopped
- 1 tablespoon of Olive oil
- 1 tablespoon of Lemon juice
- 1/2 teaspoon of Garlic powder
- 1/2 teaspoon of Sea salt
- 1/4 teaspoon of Black pepper
- 6 cups of Cucumber, chopped
- 1 Red onion, thinly sliced

Directions:

1. Combine the dill, sour cream, olive oil, garlic powder, and lemon juice in a bowl. Season the mixture with black pepper and sea salt.

2. Add in the red onions and chopped cucumbers. Serve.

Nutrition:

Servings: one cup

Calories: 86

Protein: 2g

Fat: 6g

Carbohydrates: 7g

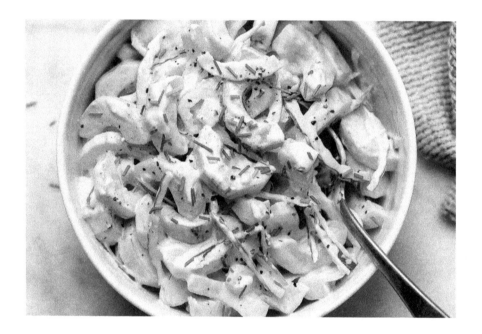

Classic Low Carb Cobb Salad

Preparation Time: 30 minutes

Cooking Time: 10 minutes

Servings: 6

Ingredients:

- 1/4 cup of red wine vinegar

- 2 teaspoons of salt

- 1 teaspoon of lemon juice

- 1 clove of garlic, minced

- 3/4 teaspoon of coarsely ground pepper

- 3/4 teaspoon of Worcestershire sauce

- 1/4 teaspoon of sugar

- 1/4 teaspoon of ground mustard

- 3/4 cup of canola oil

- 1/4 cup of olive oil

For Salad:

- 6-1/2 cups of torn romaine

- 2-1/2 cups of torn curly endive

- 1 bunch of watercress, trimmed, divided

- 2 chicken breasts, cooked, chopped

- 2 tomatoes, seeded and chopped

- 1 ripe avocado, peeled and chopped

- 3 boiled large eggs, chopped

- 1/2 cup of crumbled blue or Roquefort cheese

- 6 cooked bacon strips, crumbled

- 2 tablespoons of minced fresh chives

Directions:

1. Puree the first eight Ingredients in the blender, while adding in olive and canola oils until smooth.

2. Mix the endive, romaine, and half of watercress in a bowl. Transfer to a platter, then assemble the tomatoes, chicken, eggs, avocado, bacon, and cheese on the greens.

3. Top with chives and rest of the watercress. Drizzle one cup of dressing over the salad. serve.

Nutrition:

Servings: 1

Calories: 577

Protein:20g

Fat:52g

Carbohydrates: 10g

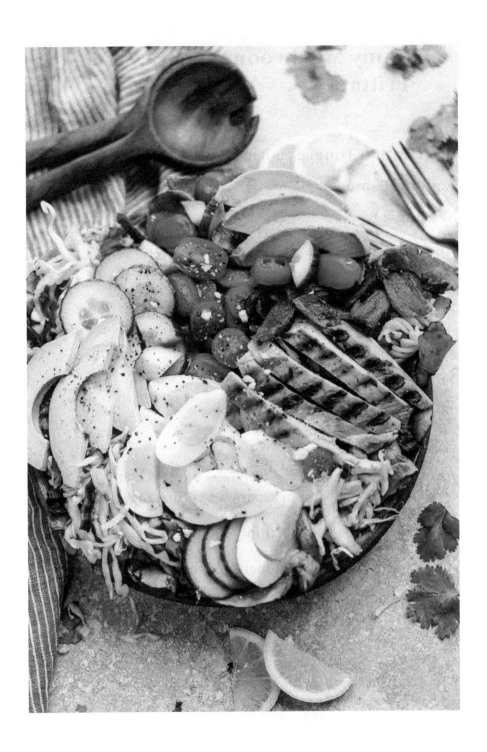

Yummy Mushroom Asparagus Frittata

Preparation Time: 25 minutes

Cooking Time: 20 minutes

Servings: 8

Ingredients:

- 8 eggs

- 1/2 cup of whole-milk ricotta cheese

- 2 tablespoons of lemon juice

- 1/2 teaspoon of salt

- 1/4 teaspoon of pepper

- 1 tablespoon of olive oil

- 1 package of frozen asparagus spears, thawed

- 1 onion, halved and thinly sliced

- 1/4 cup of baby portobello mushrooms, sliced

- 1/2 cup of sweet green or red pepper, finely chopped

Directions:

1. First, preheat the oven to about 350 degrees F, then whisk the ricotta cheese, eggs, salt, lemon juice, and pepper in a bowl.

2. Pour oil into a skillet and add in onion, asparagus, mushrooms, and red pepper. Cook until pepper and onions are tender, about eight minutes.

3. Add in the egg mixture and transfer to the oven. Bake until eggs are set, about twenty five minutes.

4. Keep aside to cool, then cut into wedges.

Nutrition:

Servings: one wedge

calories: 130

protein: 9g

fat: 8g

Carbohydrates: 5g

Special Almond Cereal

Preparation Time: 5 minutes

Cooking Time: 5 minutes

Servings: 1

Ingredients:

- 2 tablespoons almonds; chopped.

- 1/3 cup coconut milk

- 1 tablespoon chia seeds

- 2 tablespoon pepitas; roasted

- A handful blueberries

- 1 small banana; chopped.

- 1/3 cup water

Directions:

1. In a bowl, mix chia seeds with coconut milk and leave aside for 5 minutes

2. In your food processor, mix half of the pepitas with almonds and pulse them well.

3. Add this to chia seeds mix.

4. Also add the water and stir.

5. Top with the rest of the pepitas, banana pieces and blueberries and serve

Nutrition:

Calories: 200

Fat: 3

Fiber: 2

Carbs: 5

Protein: 4

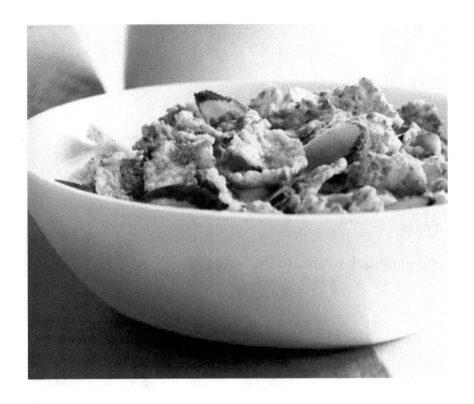

Awesome Avocado Muffins

Preparation Time: 10 minutes

Cooking Time: 20 minutes

Servings: 12

Ingredients:

- 6 bacon slices; chopped.

- 1 yellow onion; chopped.

- 1/2 teaspoon baking soda

- 1/2 cup coconut flour

- 1 cup coconut milk

- 2 cups avocado; pitted, peeled and chopped.

- 4 eggs

- Salt and black pepper to the taste.

Directions:

1. Heat up a pan, add onion and bacon; stir and brown for a few minutes

2. In a bowl, mash avocado pieces with a fork and whisk well with the eggs

3. Add milk, salt, pepper, baking soda and coconut flour and stir everything.

4. Add bacon mix and stir again.

5. Add coconut oil to muffin tray, divide eggs and avocado mix into the tray, heat oven at 350 degrees F and bake for 20 minutes

6. Divide muffins between plates and serve them for breakfast.

Nutrition:

Calories: 200

Fat: 7

Fiber: 4

Carbs: 7

Protein: 5

Tasty WW Pancakes

Preparation Time: 12 minutes

Cooking Time: 3 minutes

Servings: 4

Ingredients:

- 2 ounces' cream cheese

- 1 teaspoon stevia

- 1/2 teaspoon cinnamon; ground

- 2 eggs

- Cooking spray

Directions:

1. Mix the eggs with the cream cheese, stevia, and cinnamon in a blender, and mix well.

2. Heat pan with cooking spray over medium high heat. add 1/4 of the batter, spread well, cook 2 minutes, invert and cook 1 minute more

3. Move to a plate and repeat with the rest of the dough.

4. Serve them right away.

Nutrition:

Calories: 344

Fat: 23

Fiber: 12

Carbs: 3

Protein: 16

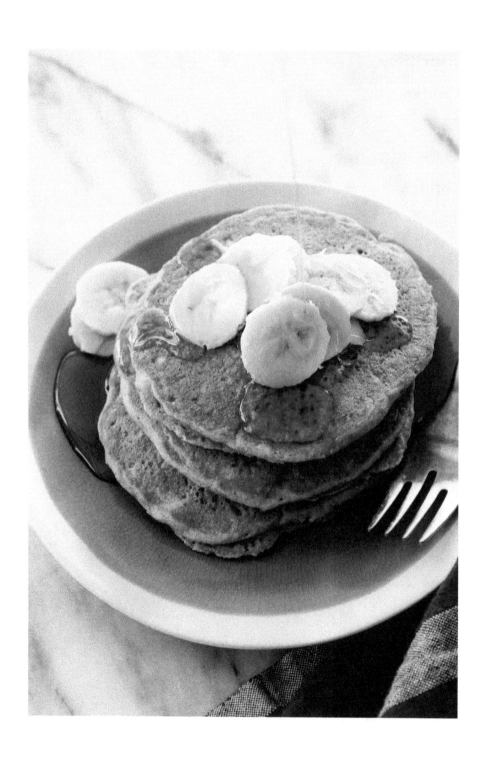

Dinner

Air Fryer Fish And Chips

Servings: 4

Cooking Time: 35 Mints

Ingredients:

- 4 cups of any fish fillet

- flour: 1/4 cup

- Whole wheat breadcrumbs: one cup

- One egg

- Oil: 2 tbsp.

- Potatoes

- Salt: 1 tsp.

Directions:

1. Cut the potatoes in fries. Then coat with oil and salt.

2. Cook in the air fryer for 20 minutes at 400 F, toss the fries halfway through.

3. In the meantime, coat fish in flour, then in the whisked egg, and finally in breadcrumbs mix.

4. Place the fish in the air fryer and let it cook at 330F for 15 minutes.

5. Flip it halfway through, if needed.

6. Serve with tartar sauce and salad green.

Nutrition:

Calories: 409kcal

Carbohydrates: 44g

Protein: 30g

Fat: 11g

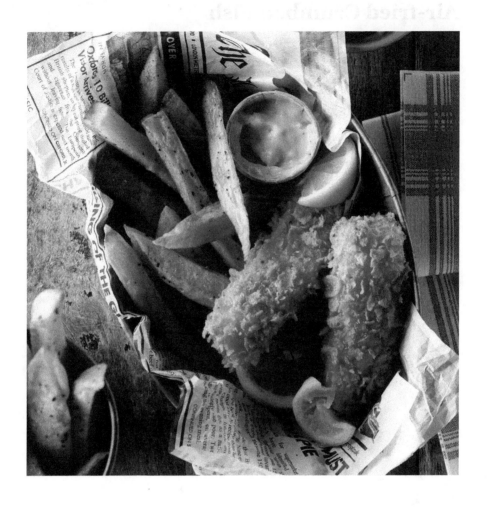

Air-fried Crumbed Fish

Servings: 2

Cooking Time: 12 Mints

Ingredients:

- Four fish fillets

- Olive oil: 4 tablespoons

- One egg beaten

- Whole wheat breadcrumbs: ¼ cup

Directions:

1. Let the air fryer preheat to 180 C.

2. In a bowl, mix breadcrumbs with oil. Mix well

3. First, coat the fish in the egg mix (egg mix with water) then in the breadcrumb mix. Coat well

4. Place in the air fryer, let it cook for 10-12 minutes.

5. Serve hot with salad green and lemon.

Nutrition:

Calories: 254 Cal

Fat: 12.7g

Carbohydrates: 10.2g

protein: 15.5g

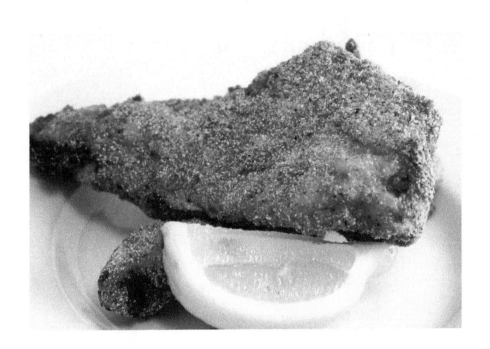

Air Fryer Lemon Garlic Shrimp

Servings: 2

Cooking Time: 10 Mints

Ingredients:

- Olive oil: 1 Tbsp.

- Small shrimp: 4 cups, peeled, tails removed

- One lemon juice and zest

- Parsley: 1/4 cup sliced

- Red pepper flakes(crushed): 1 pinch

- Four cloves of grated garlic

- Sea salt: 1/4 teaspoon

Directions:

1. Let air fryer heat to 400F

2. Mix olive oil, lemon zest, red pepper flakes, shrimp, kosher salt, and garlic in a bowl and coat the shrimp well.

3. Place shrimps in the air fryer basket, coat with oil spray.

4. Cook at 400 F for 8 minutes. Toss the shrimp halfway through

5. Serve with lemon slices and parsley.

Nutrition:

Cal 140

Fat: 18g

Net Carbs: 8g

Protein: 20g

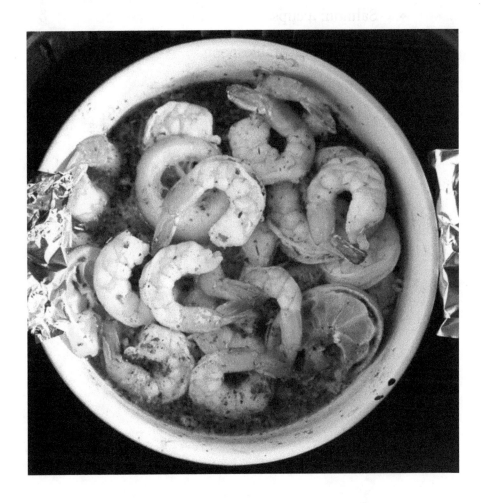

Quick & Easy Air Fryer Salmon

Servings: 4

Cooking Time: 12 Mints

Ingredients:

- Lemon pepper seasoning: 2 teaspoons

- Salmon: 4 cups

- Olive oil: one tablespoon

- Seafood seasoning:2 teaspoons

- Half lemon's juice

- Garlic powder:1 teaspoon

- Kosher salt to taste

Directions:

1. In a bowl, add one tbsp. of olive oil and half lemon's juice.

2. Pour this mixture over salmon and rub. Leave the skin on salmon. It will come off when cooked.

3. Rub the salmon with kosher salt and spices.

4. Put parchment paper in the air fryer basket. Put the salmon in the air fryer.

5. Cook at 360 F for ten minutes. Cook until inner salmon temperature reaches 140 F.

6. Let the salmon rest five minutes before serving.

7. Serve with salad greens and lemon wedges.

Nutrition:

Cal: 132

total fat: 7.4g

carbohydrates: 12 g

protein: 22.1g

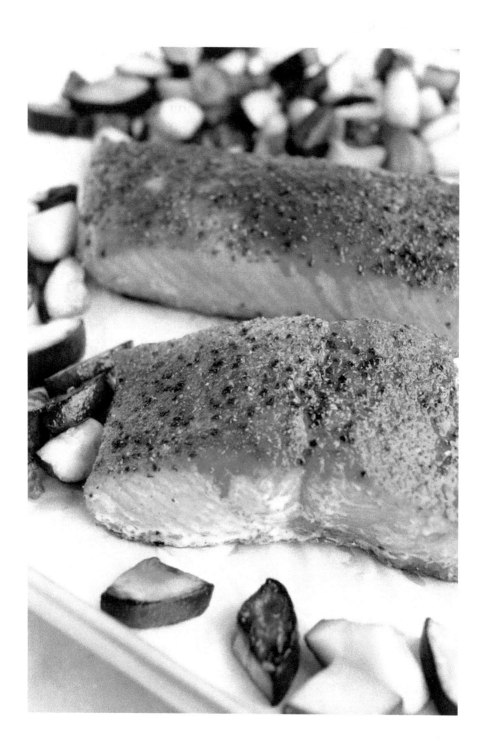

Shrimp Spring Rolls

Servings: 4

Cooking Time: 25 Mints

Ingredients:

- Deveined raw shrimp: half cup chopped(peeled)

- Olive oil: 2 and 1/2 tbsp.

- Matchstick carrots: 1 cup

- Slices of red bell pepper: 1 cup

- Red pepper: 1/4 teaspoon(crushed)

- Slices of snow peas: 3/4 cup

- Shredded cabbage: 2 cups

- Lime juice: 1 tablespoon

- Sweet chili sauce: half cup

- Fish sauce: 2 teaspoons

- Eight spring roll(wrappers)

Directions:

1. In a skillet, add one and a half tbsp. of olive, until smoking lightly. Stir in bell pepper, cabbage, carrots, and cook for two minutes. Turn off the heat, take out in a dish and cool for five minutes.

2. In a bowl, add shrimp, lime juice, cabbage mixture, crushed red pepper, fish sauce, and snow peas. Mix well

3. Lay spring roll wrappers on a plate. Add 1/4 cup of filling in the middle of each wrapper. Fold tightly with water. Brush the olive oil over folded rolls.

4. Put spring rolls in the air fryer basket and cook for 6 to 7 minutes at 390°F until light brown and crispy.

5. You may serve with sweet chili sauce.

Nutrition:

Calories 180

Fat 9g

Protein 17g

Carbohydrate 9g

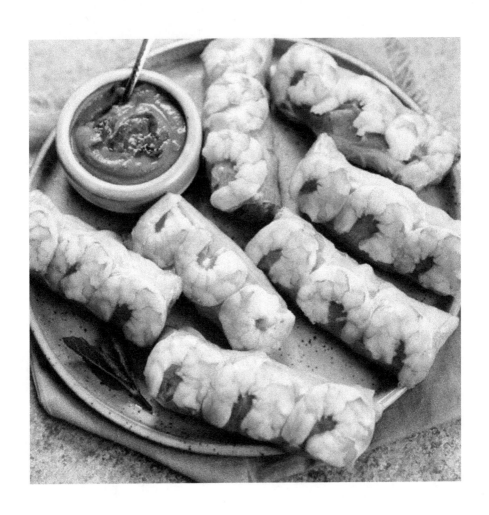

South West Tortilla Crusted Tilapia Salad

Servings: 2

Cooking Time: 15 Mints

Ingredients:

- Tilapia fillets (Tortilla Crusted)

- Mixed greens: six cups

- Chipotle Lime Dressing: half cup

- Diced red onion: 1/3 cup

- One avocado

- Cherry tomatoes: one cup

Directions:

1. On frozen tilapia fillet, spray the olive oil.

2. Put in the air fryer basket, cook at 390° for 15-18 minutes.

3. In a bowl, add tomatoes, red onion, and half of the greens. Coat with the Chipotle Lime Dressing.

4. Serve the fish with vegetables.

Nutrition:

Cal: 260

total fat: 19g

carbohydrates: 7.6g

protein: 19.2g

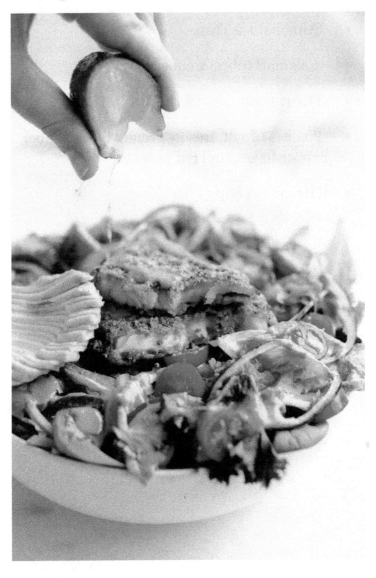

Sriracha & Honey Tossed Calamari

Servings: 2

Cooking Time: 20 Mints

Ingredients:

- Club soda: 1 cup

- Sriracha: 1-2 Tbsp.

- Calamari tubes: 2 cups

- Flour: 1 cup

- Pinches of salt, freshly ground black pepper, red pepper flakes, and red pepper

- Honey: 1/2 cup

Directions:

1.   Cut the calamari tubes into rings. Submerge them with club soda. Let it rest for ten minutes.

2.   In the meantime, in a bowl, add freshly ground black pepper, flour, red pepper, and kosher salt and mix well.

3.   Drain the calamari and pat dry with a paper towel. Coat well the calamari in the flour mix and set aside.

4.   Spray oil in the air fryer basket and put calamari in one single layer.

5.   Cook at 375 for 11 minutes. Toss the rings twice while cooking. Meanwhile, to make sauce honey, red pepper flakes, and sriracha in a bowl, well.

6.   Take calamari out from the basket, mix with sauce cook for another two minutes more. Serve with salad green.

Nutrition:

Cal 252

Fat: 38g

Carbs: 3.1g

Protein: 41g

Air Fryer Shrimp Tacos

Servings: 4

Cooking Time: 10 Mints

Ingredients:

- Flour tortillas: 12

- Avocado sliced: 1 cup

- Chipotle chili powder: 1 tsp

- Raw jumbo shrimp: 24 pieces, deveined, peeled, without tail

- Smoked paprika: 1/2 tsp

- Salt: 1/4 tsp

- Olive oil: 1 tbsp.

- Green salsa: ½ cup

- Light brown sugar: 1 and 1/2 tsp

- Garlic powder: 1/2 tsp

- Low-fat sour cream: 1/2 cup

- Red onion: 1/2 cup diced

Directions:

1. Let the oven preheat to 400 F and spray the air fryer basket with oil spray.

2. In a bowl, mix chipotle chili powder, salt, brown sugar, smoked paprika, and garlic powder, mix well

3. Pat dry the shrimp, put shrimp in zip lock bag and add the seasonings and toss to coat well

4. Place shrimp in air fryer basket in one even layer, cook for four minutes and flip them overcook for four minutes more

5. For the sauce, mix sour cream and green salsa.

6. Put shrimp in a tortilla, top with sauce, shrimp, red onion, sliced avocado serve with lime wedges.

Nutrition:

Cal 228

Fat: 18

carbs: 16 g

Protein: 20 g

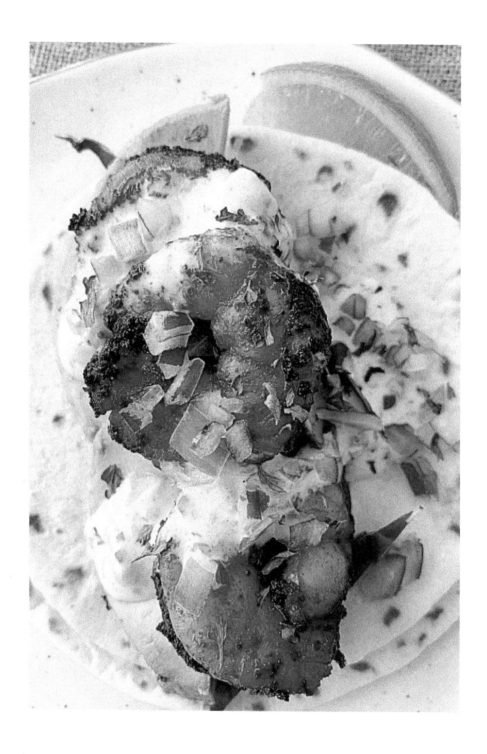

Index Recipes:

CPSIA information can be obtained
at www.ICGtesting.com
Printed in the USA
BVHW012329150321
602550BV00005B/595